AF488035

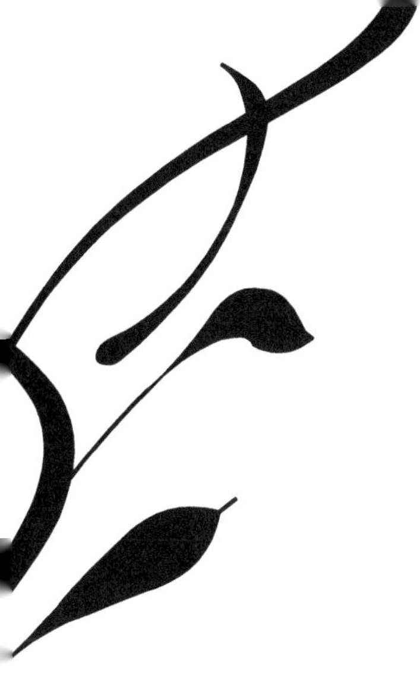

We are Each of Us Beautiful

Written and Illustrated by Lindsey K. Frazier

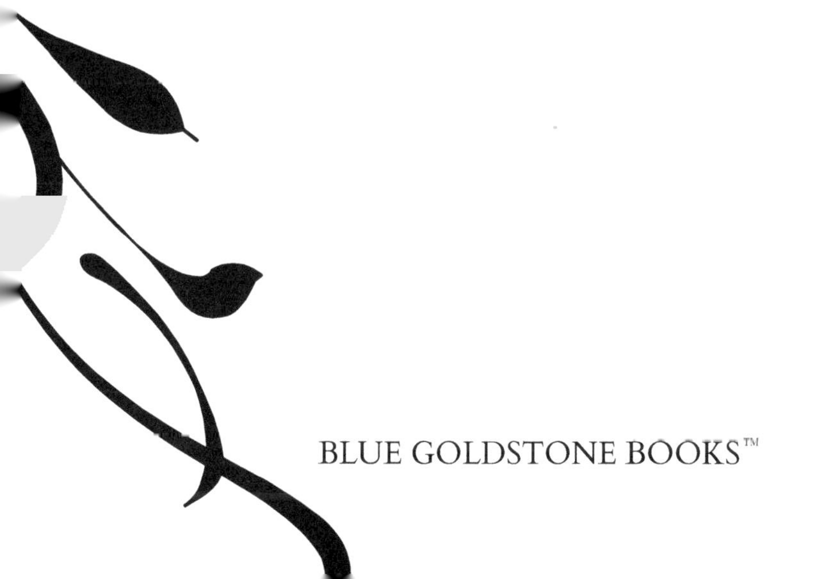

BLUE GOLDSTONE BOOKS™

To my beautiful sisters

We are Each of Us Beautiful

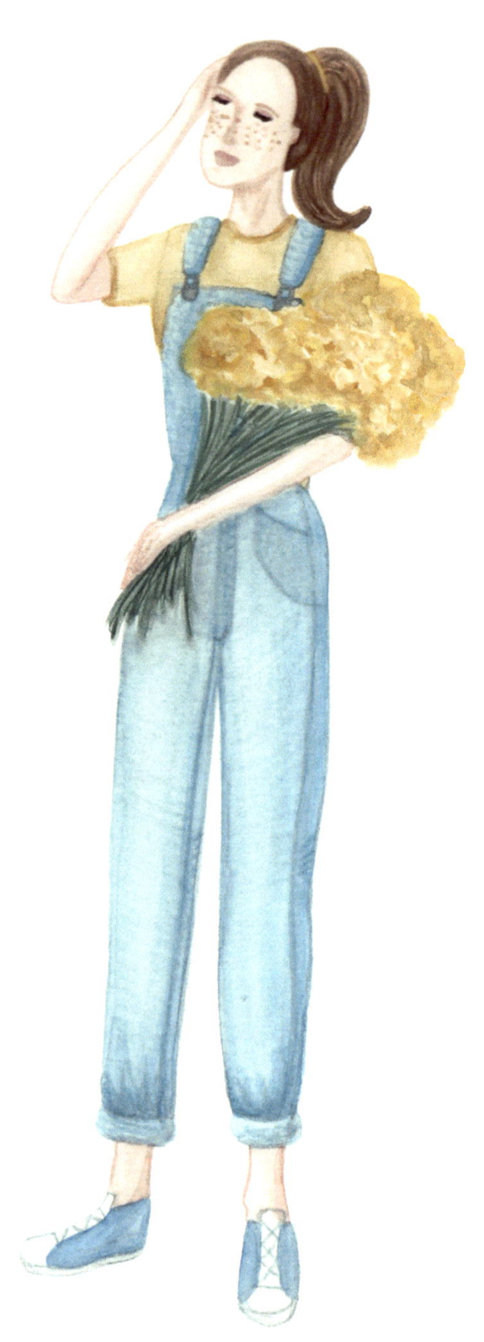

We are each of us beautiful,

Like flowers growing in a garden,

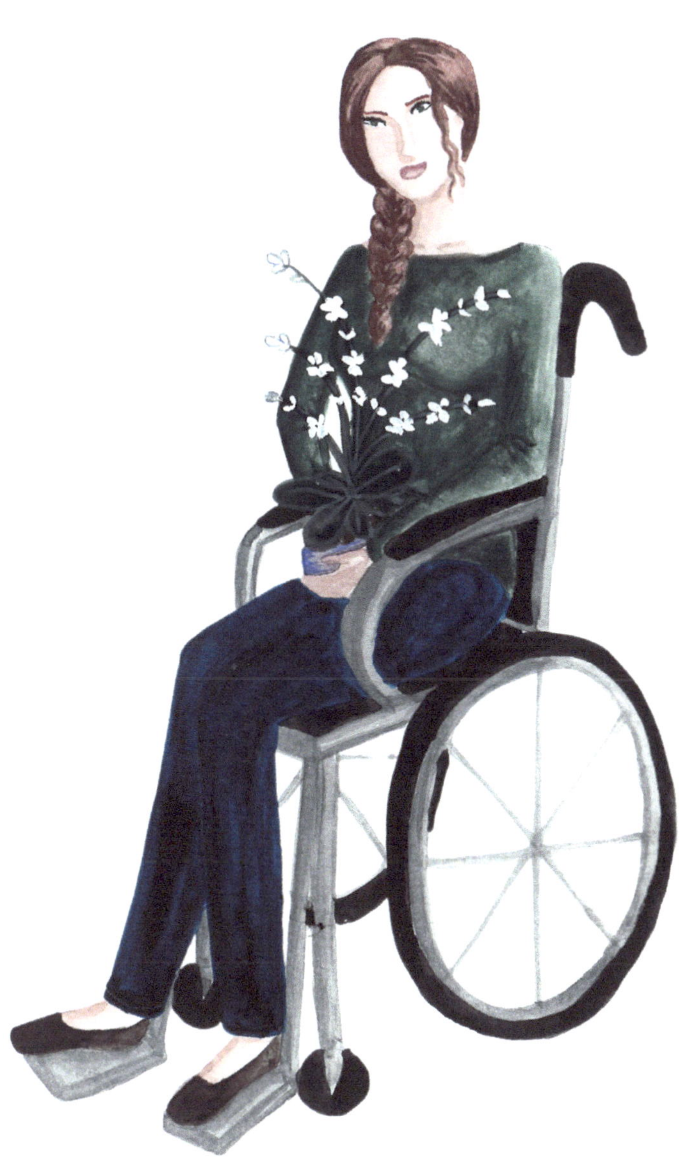

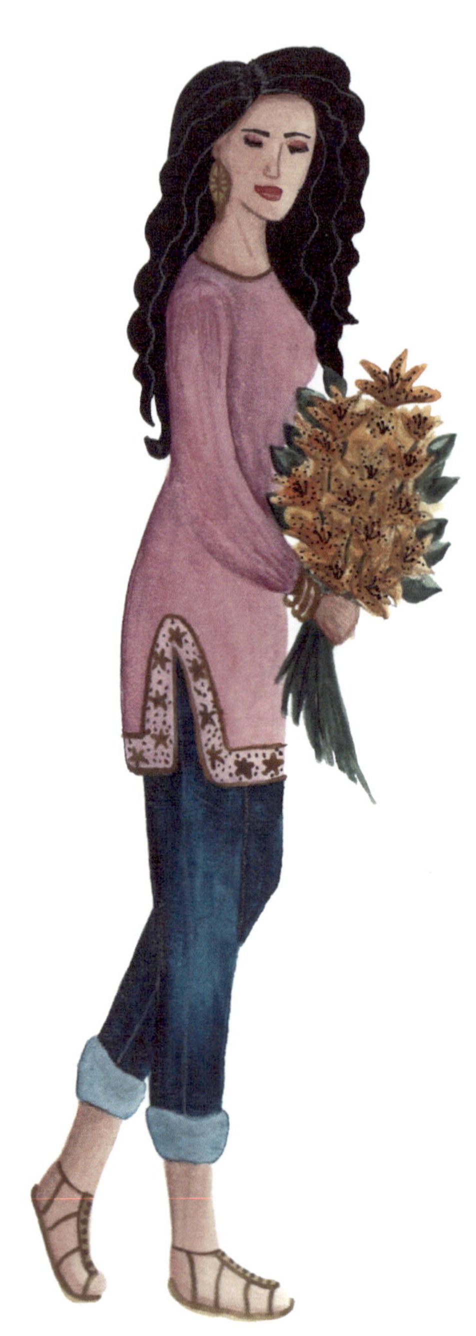

Each representative
of a different kind of
beauty.

-8-

Flowers come in a variety of colors, shapes, and sizes,

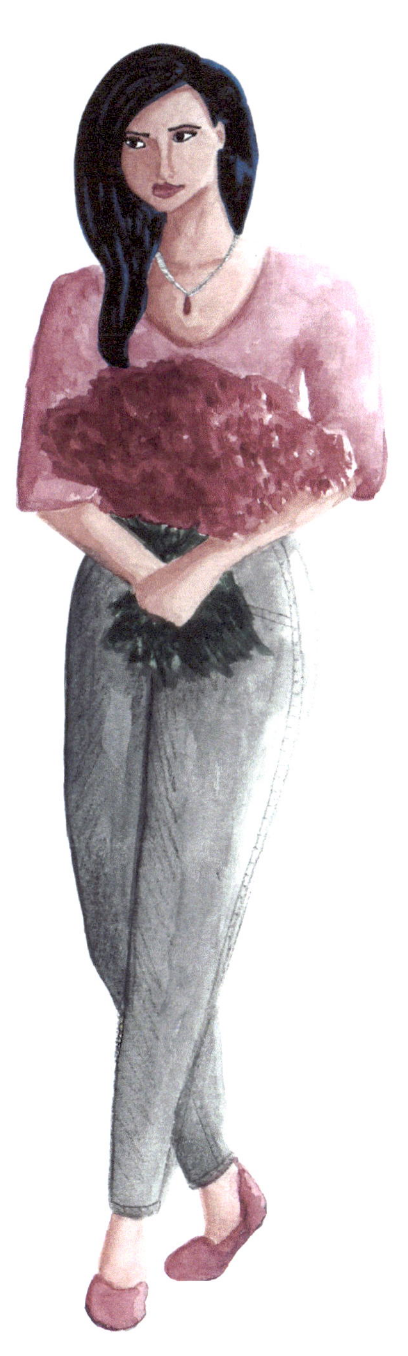

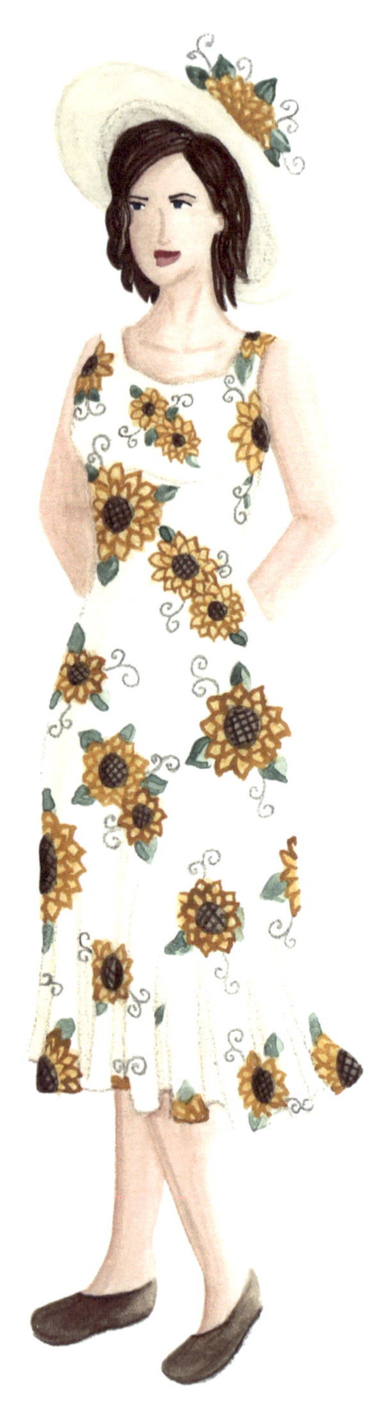

From bright yellow sunflowers,

To small and delicate forget-me-nots.

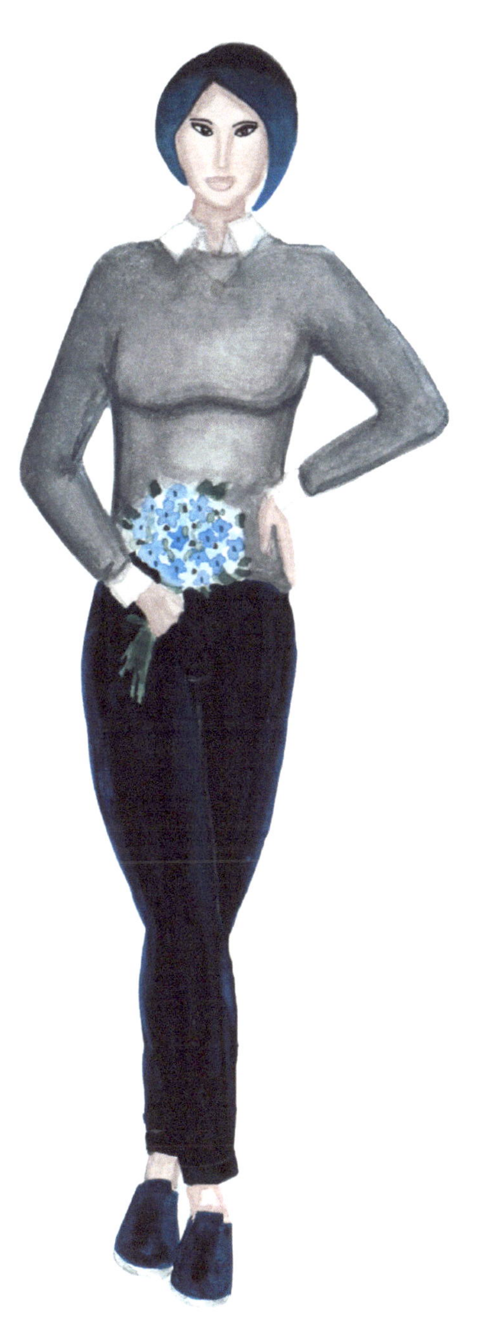

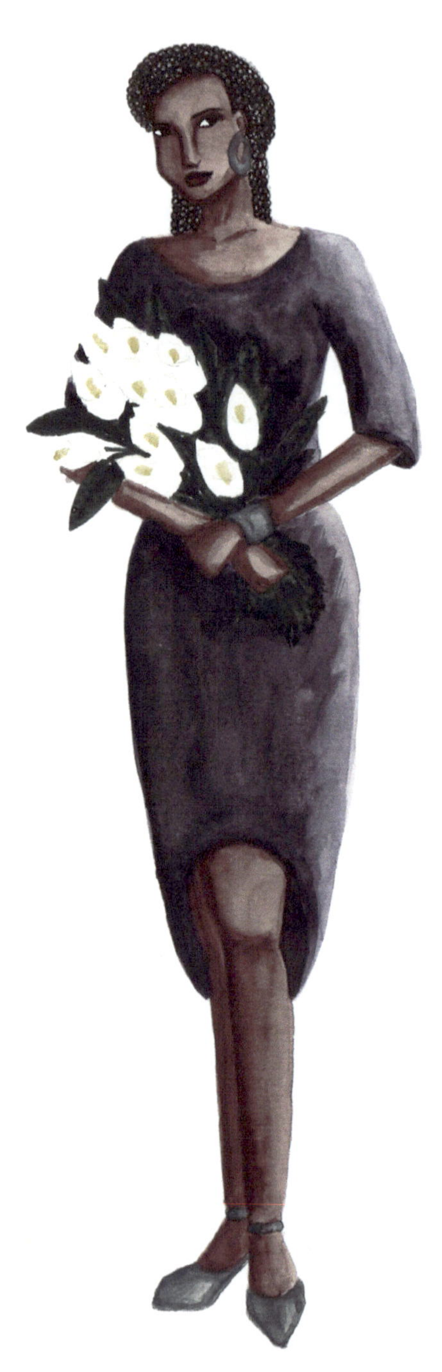

One flower does not
compare itself to another.

Instead, it grows

confidently,

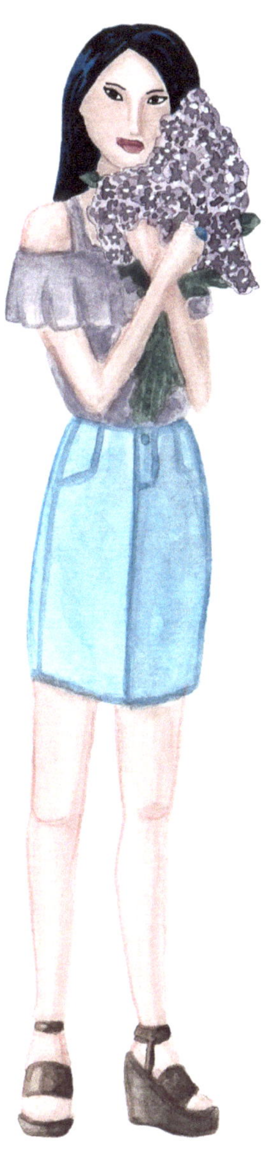

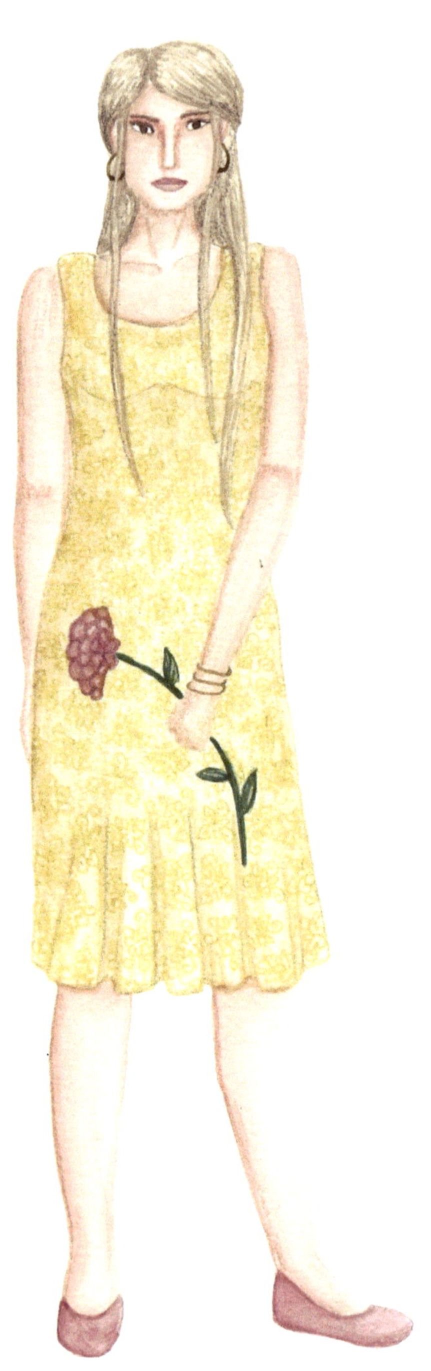

Anchoring its roots
firmly into the soil,

-20-

Stretching its petals gracefully to the sky.

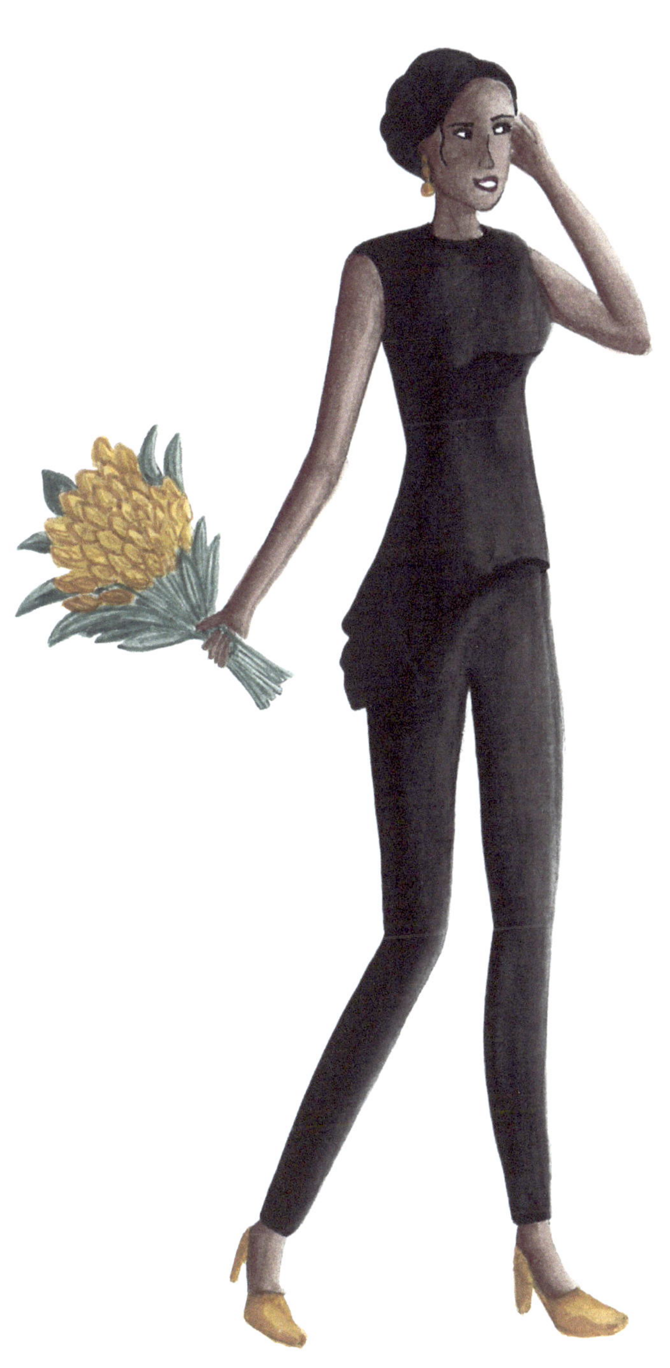

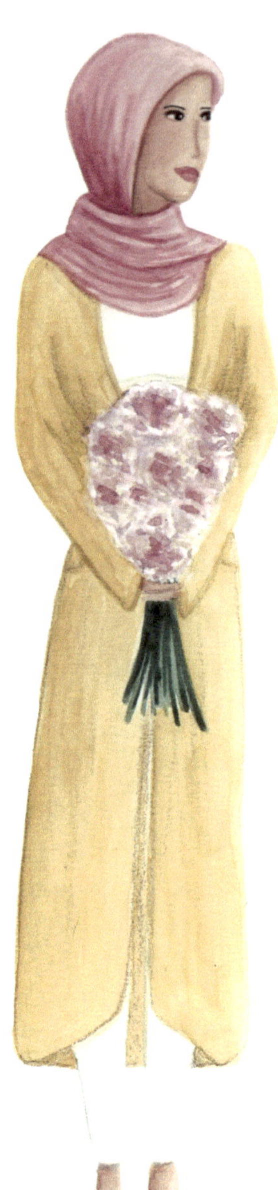

Each makes the world a
little brighter,

Each makes the world a bit sweeter.

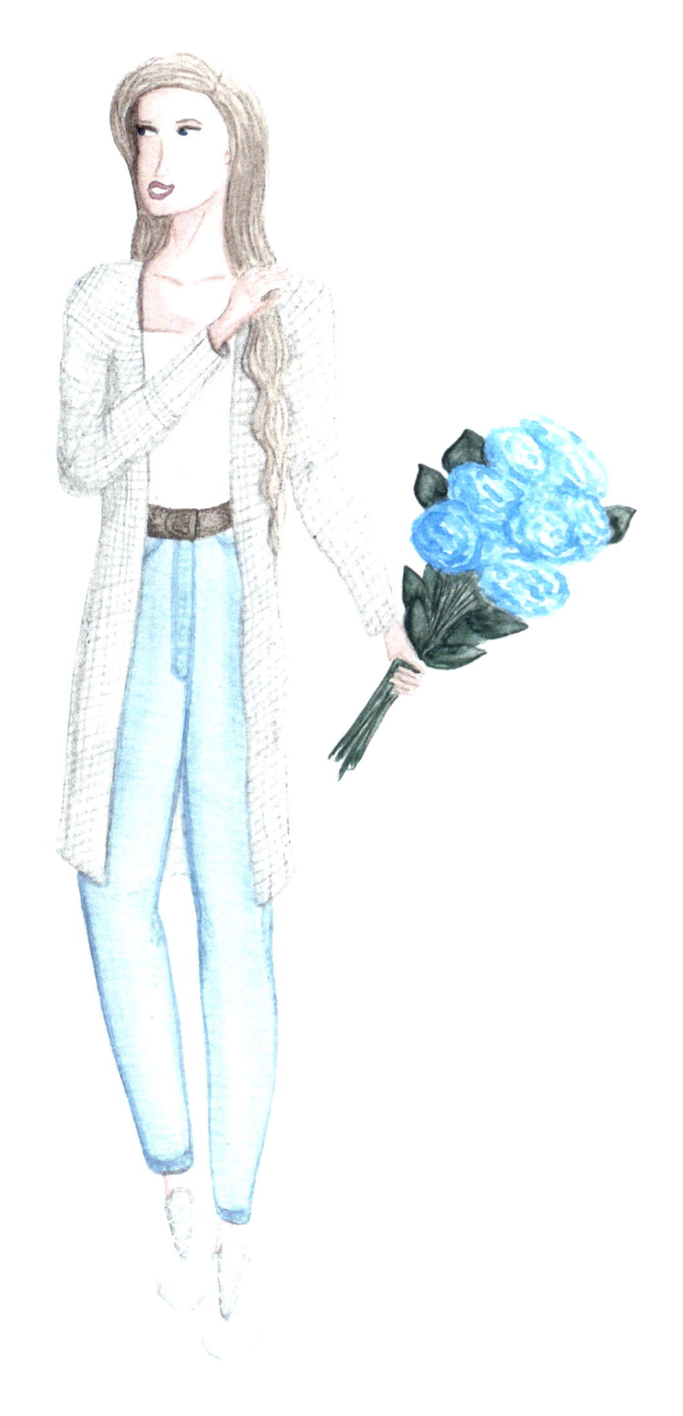

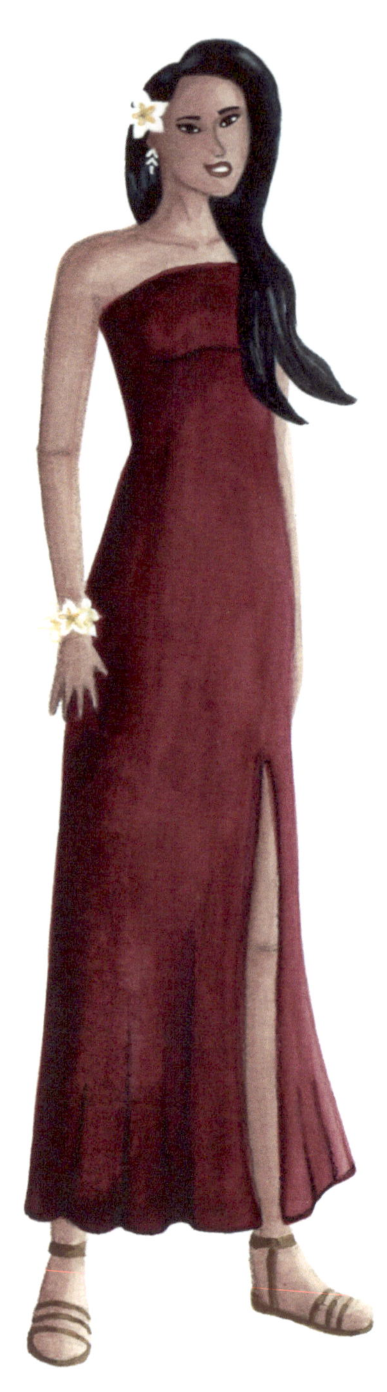

-27-

We can emulate the
flowers,

Growing confident and
strong,

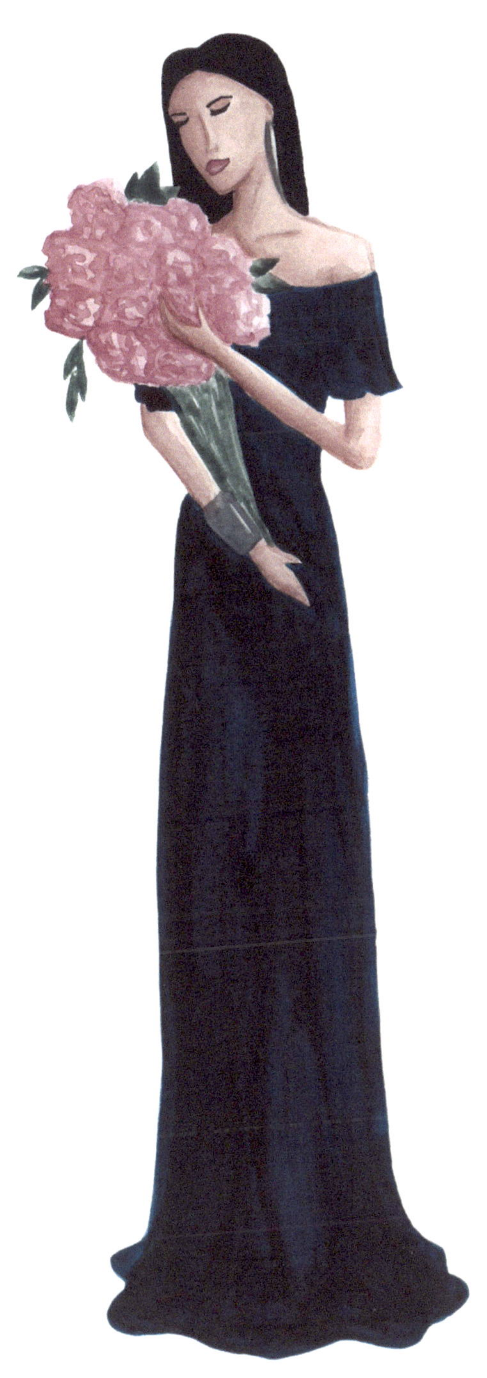

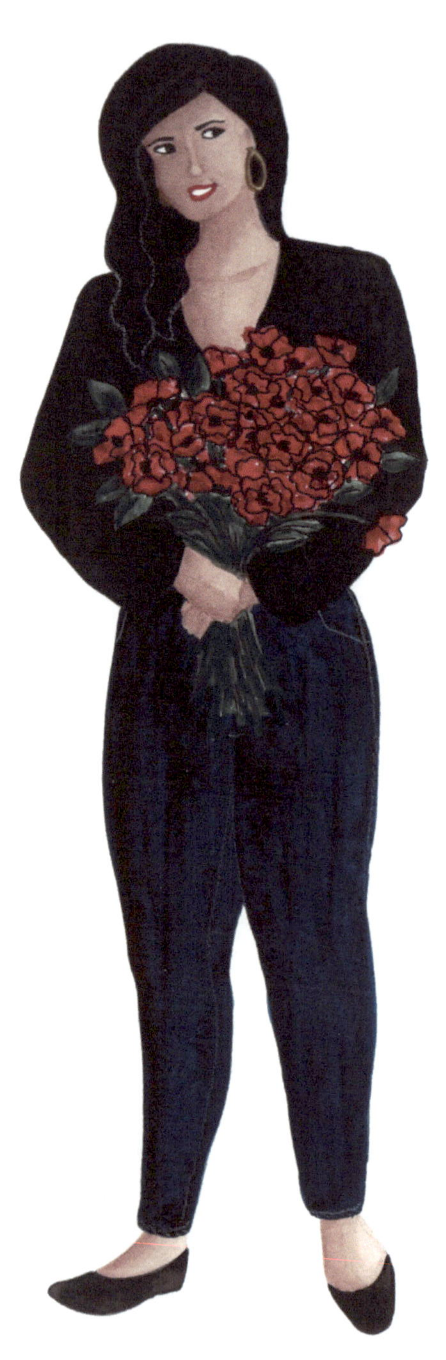

Lighting up the world
with our individual
beauty,

-32-

For we are each of us
beautiful,

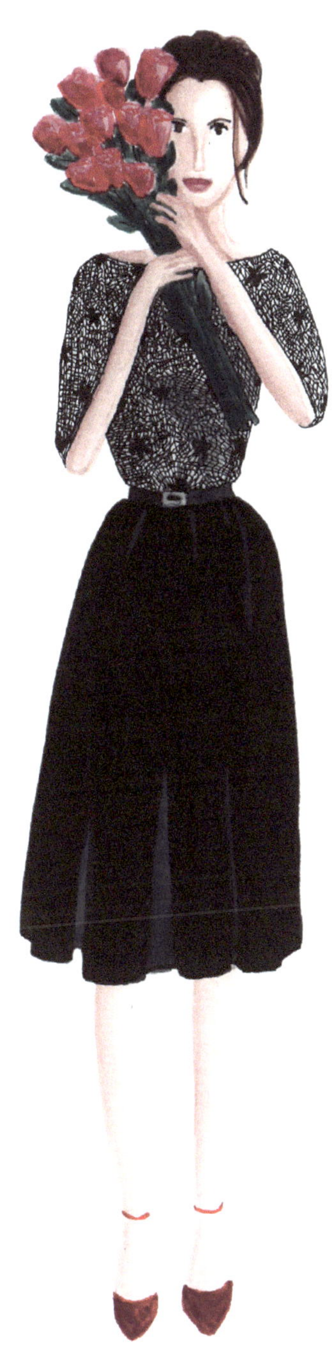

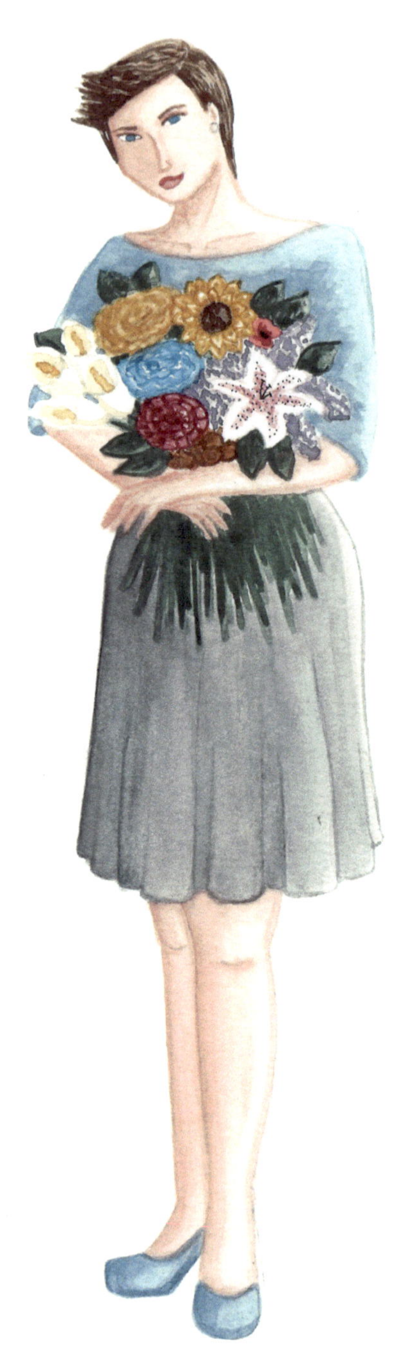

-35-

Just as we are.

Author's Note

No matter what you look like, you have probably experienced a time when you did not feel beautiful. I certainly have had those days. It is hard to feel beautiful when you are constantly bombarded by social media that tells you you must look a certain way in order to be desirable. Even when you finally achieve those 'desirable' traits, you don't necessarily feel like you are enough. It's an awful feeling, one I have struggled with for years. Until I began to think of myself as a flower.

There are hundreds of thousands of different species of flowers in the world—isn't that amazing? And each one is unique and beautiful. Do you have a favorite flower? Mine is a pink peony. Red roses are often considered to be the most 'perfect' and 'beautiful' flowers, and while I certainly like red roses, pink peonies are still my favorite. Someone decided red roses equal 'perfection', but that does not mean that all other flowers are inferior—it's all about our preference. We do not shame flowers for not looking like roses—we appreciate the individual beauty each flower has to offer. The elegant beauty of a peony, the bright beauty of a sunflower, the cheerful beauty of a daisy, or the wild beauty of a poppy. All those flowers are gorgeous! People are the same way. They all display a different type of beauty, and it is about time we recognize them for it.

I hope you will continue to celebrate the unique beauty of those around you in your day to day life, as well as remind yourself of your own amazing beauty every time you look in the mirror.

Remember that you are beautiful just as you are.

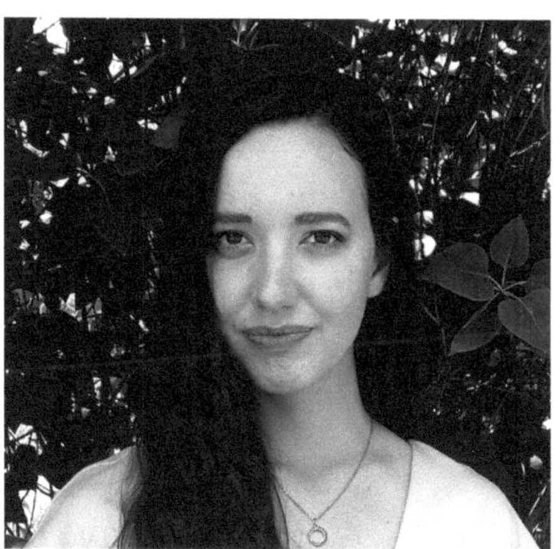

About the Author

Lindsey K. Frazier earned a Multidisciplinary Studies degree with a Certificate in Leadership from Boise State University, where she studied art, history, and leadership practices. When she isn't writing or working through her never-ending reading list, she enjoys dancing, watercolor painting, and going on walks.

Instagram: lindseykfrazier
Website: lindseykfrazier.com
YouTube: Lindsey K. Frazier

www.ingramcontent.com/pod-product-compliance
Lightning Source LLC
Chambersburg PA
CBHW040747110726
47973CB00013B/199